# Rooter Can't Breathe

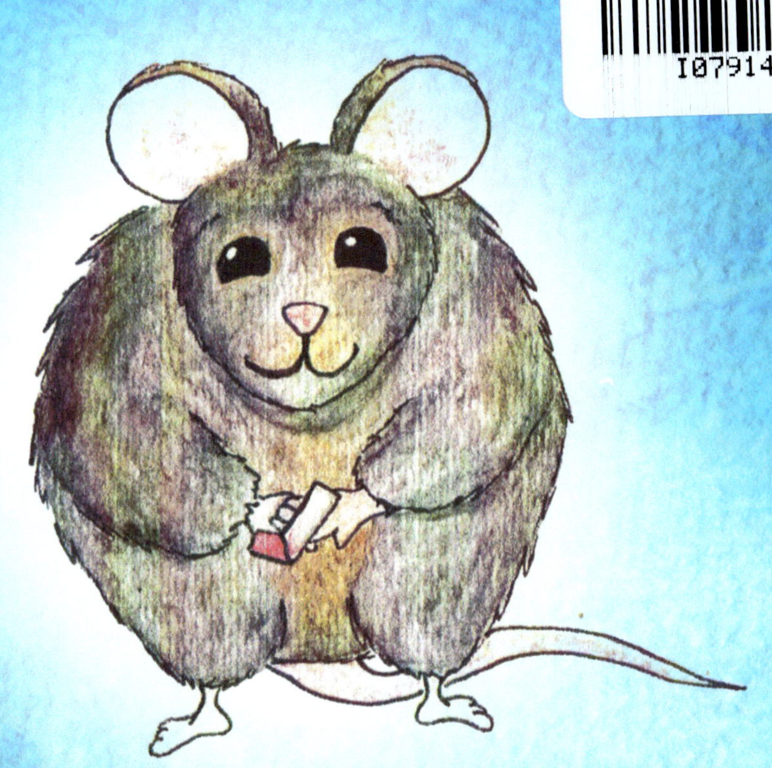

## Cindi Hoiness RN

Illustrator: Blake Morgan, Editors: Jonatha Elenburg and Leslie Hittmeier

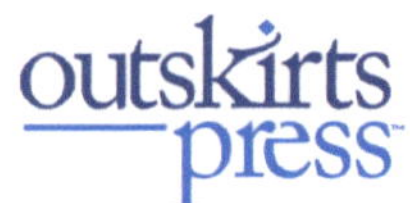

This Book Belongs to:

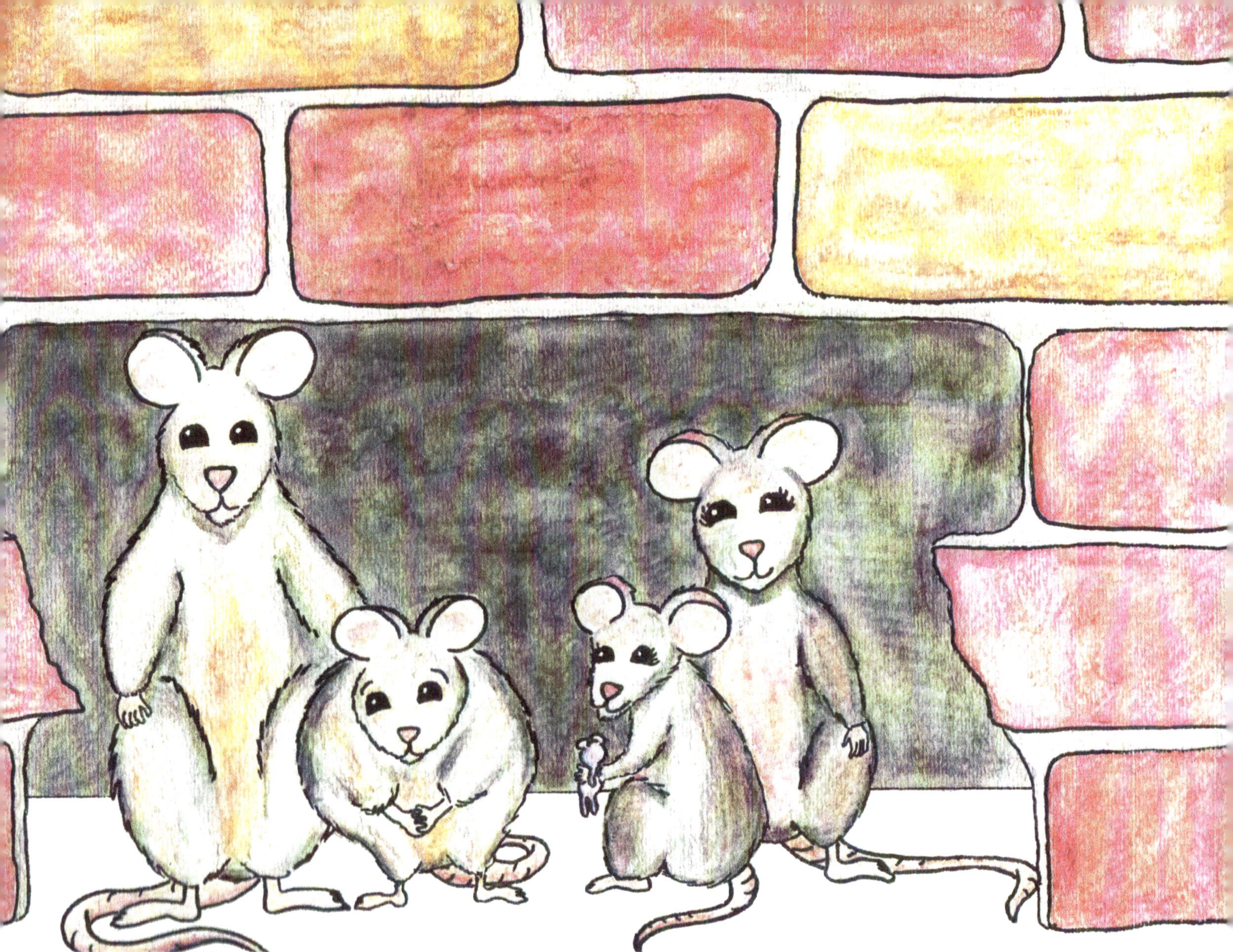

# Chapter 1

This is a story about Rooter. He is a pack rat. He lives in a smelly, air-polluted town called Smogville.

Rooter comes from a long line of the best, top-notch, sneaky pack rats in the west. He has a dad named Snooter. His mom is named Cattera and his sister is named Rattella. They all live together in a large cozy nest filled with shiny objects from all of Snooter's sneaky treasure hunts.

# Chapter 2

Rooter loves to play outside and his most favorite game in the whole world is "Catch the Gobblygook".

In case you don't know how to play Gobblygook, let me tell you. It is like a game of Tag which requires great speed, and you must have a hideous, scary look on your face! You know, the kind of look you get when you smell stinky, dirty socks! Ewheeew!!

One day Rooter and his friends decided they wanted to have the biggest game of Gobblygook ever to be played! So they called out to everyone they knew and told them to spread the word. All who want to play are to meet at the Smogville field at high noon.

# Chapter 3

Its finally high noon and hundreds of players showed up from all over town.

Rooter gathers everyone together and tells all of players to spread out away from each other. Then at that moment Sam the squirrel yells, "I'm it!" He takes off running and tags Rooter right away. Rooter yells "I'm it" and off he runs zigzagging this way and that way all over the field. He was laughing and trying to keep the scary look on his face until he noticed he was having a tough time breathing. When suddenly, Rooter drops to his knees on the ground! He can't breathe!

With his hands at his chest, "I...I...I can't breathe!" Rooter squeaks. Quickly Rooter's best friend, Gofer, runs to get Rooter's mom. "Cattera, Cattera! Come quick! It's Rooter! He can't breathe again!" Cattera rushes out of the nest toward Gofer and they both run very fast back to Rooter. As they get closer to Rooter, Cattera can see he is wheezing and gasping for air. Rooter's friends are trying to keep him calm but Rooter is very upset and afraid.

"Try to relax, Rooter," says Tom the cat. Cattera runs right up to Rooter. She picks him up and starts carrying him home. Cattera turns back and yells, "Please come by tomorrow. He'll be fine by then."

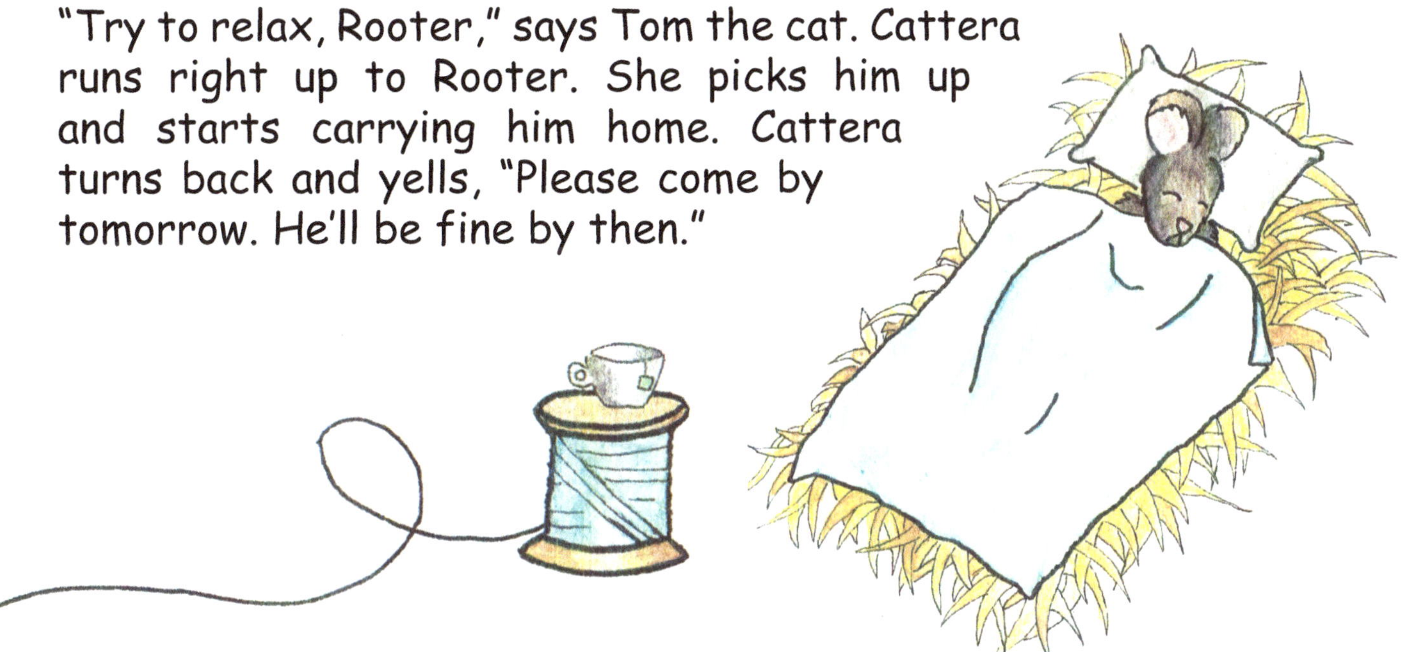

# Chapter 4

When they get home Cattera heats up some hot tea for Rooter to drink. "Here Rooter, drink this tea. It may help you breathe a little better." Rooter sips the tea, and soon Rooter starts to breathe a little better. Then he lays down for a nap.

Just then Rooter's sister, Rattella, comes bursting through the rat hole, yelling, "Mom! Where is Rooter; is he ok? Can he breathe now?"

"Shhh, honey, he's ok he is sleeping." As Cattera is rubbing Rooter's back she quietly whispers, "Rooter, I wish I knew how to help you when you can't breathe."

Rooter slowly opens his eyes. "I know, mom. It always happens when I run, I can't seem to catch my breath. I'm just not going to play anymore." He slowly closes his eyes and falls asleep.

Later that evening Rooter's dad, Snooter, comes home after a very long day of hunting. "Cattera, where are you? My eyes are killing me! They hurt so bad from all that smog, I could barely see today," says Snooter as he rubs his eyes.

# Chapter 5

"Yes, I know the smog is so thick today and Rooter had another breathing attack. I am so worried, Snooter, we must take him to see Dr. Puddlemug in the morning," sighs Cattera.

The next day they all head to Dr. Puddlemug's office. "Well, hello Snooter and Cattera. What brings you here today?" says Dr. Puddlemug.

"It's Rooter," says Cattera. "He keeps having these breathing attacks that make him wheeze and he can't seem to catch his breath. It seems to happen when he plays hard or runs," says Cattera as she looks down at Rooter and reaches to hold his hand.

"Well...let's see what's going on with Rooter," smiles Dr. Puddlemug. "Tell me, Rooter, what does it feel like when you can't breathe?"

"Well," says Rooter, "it feels like I am trying to breathe through a small straw. It's hard to breathe in and out and I make this funny wheezy sound in my chest. It really scares me."

"Hummm...I see, hummm...uhuh...yep...very interesting, yet not surprising," mumbles Dr. Puddlemug. "I have seen this before and a lot lately, unfortunately, because of the smog." He then leans into Rooter to listen to his chest. Just then Dr. Puddlemug stands up and steps back. With a strong voice he says, "I know what this is! It's asthma!"

"Asthma" says Cattera as she reaches out and hugs Rooter.

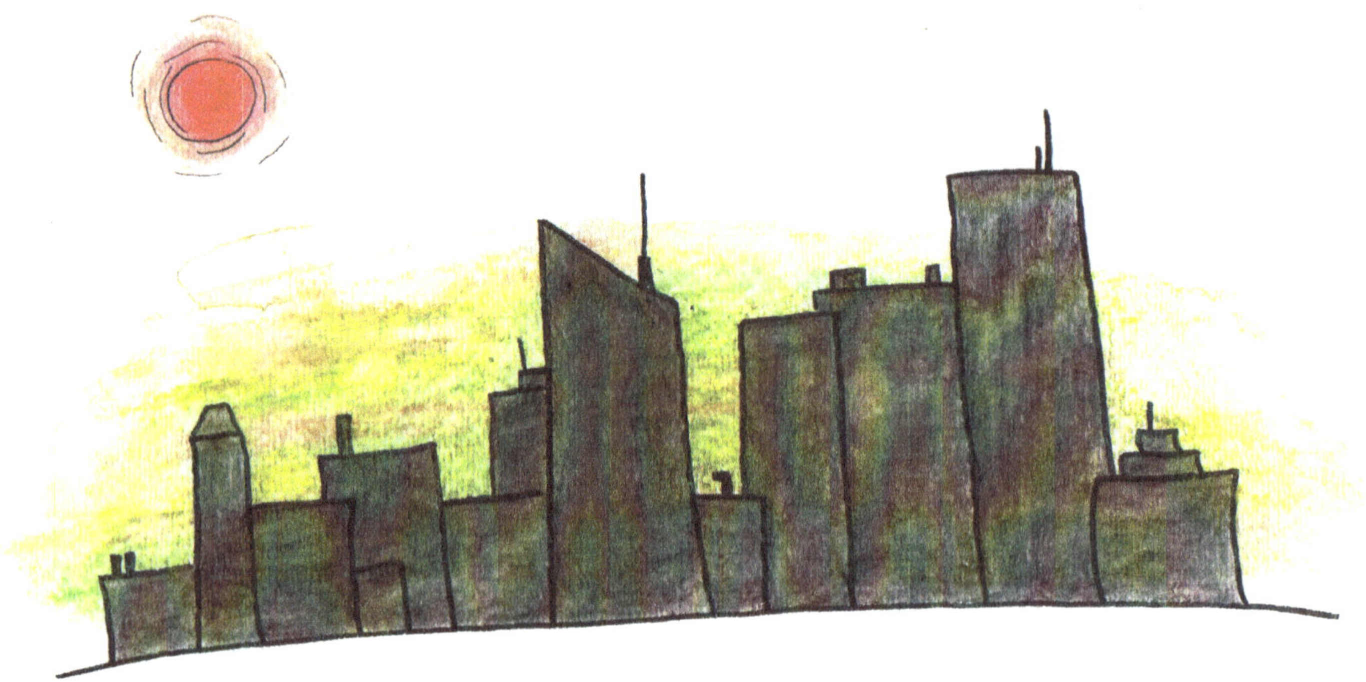

Dr. Puddlemug then turns and looks out the window where he sees layers of orange, greenish-brown haze hanging over the city of Smogville. In a low, voice he says, "Smoggville needs to clean up its air but Asthma is also caused by allergies too."

"What can we do now for Rooter when he can't breathe? Should he stop playing?" asks Cattera.

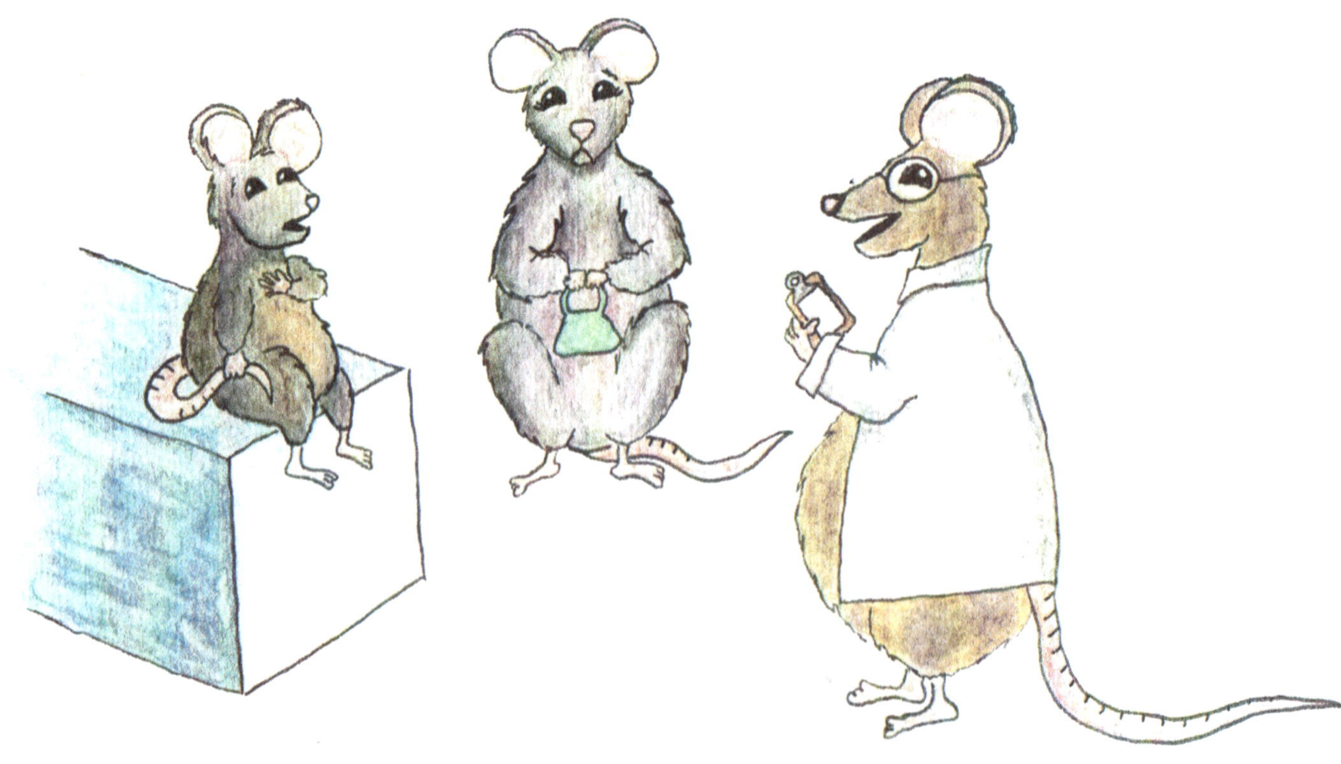

"NO! That would be bad. He needs to keep his lungs strong and healthy and the medication will help him breathe better and stay active." Dr. Puddlemug reaches over and takes a spray device off the shelf. "Here, Rooter, you use this spray before you play hard or run. Use it every time. **And I mean every time.** Do you understand, Rooter? This will help you breathe easier. Just hold it up to your mouth, breathe out and push down on the spray, then breathe in as deeply as you can." Rooter tries it and is amazed how easy it is to use. "Wow, I feel I can breathe better already," Smiles Rooter. "Thanks Dr. Puddlemug for all your help" smiles Snooter.

# Chapter 6

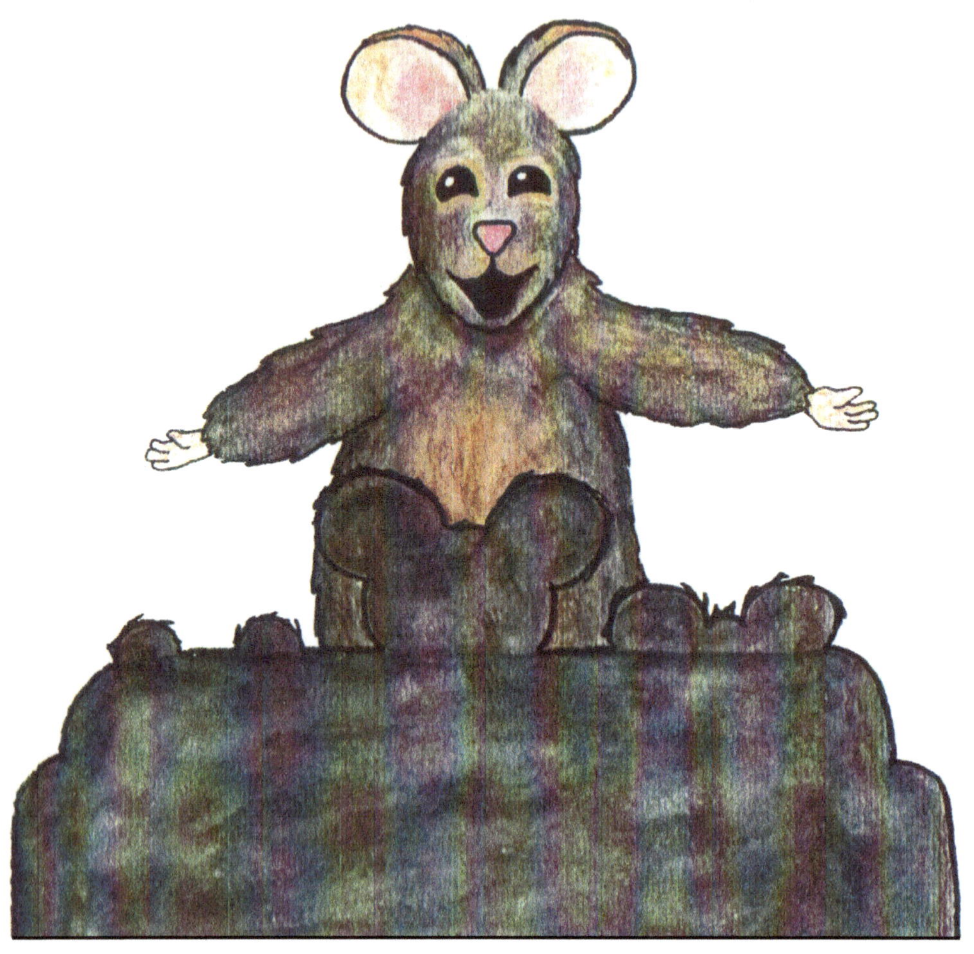

Early the next day Snooter gathers everyone up for a family meeting. "I have been thinking, and I feel it's best for the whole family to pack up and move out of Smogville today."

"What! Today!" yells Rattella. Snooter looks at Rattella.

"Yes today. Please go pack and meet me outside pronto!" Well, being pack rats it took them awhile to pack. Standing out side Snooter waits to give them his plan. "Ok, family, first we are going to catch a ride in that big trailer over there. I overheard the people that live in it, and they said they are going to a place that is in the mountains with lots of fresh air", says Snooter. Cattera moves first and leads the way with all following over to the large motorized object. Then they all jump up on the metal step. Snooter sees a hole in the door that they all can squeeze through. Once inside they quickly run to a small opening under a cabinet for safety. Within a few minutes there is a loud squeak and a huge jolt that throws them all forward against the wall. And off they go...to a new adventure!

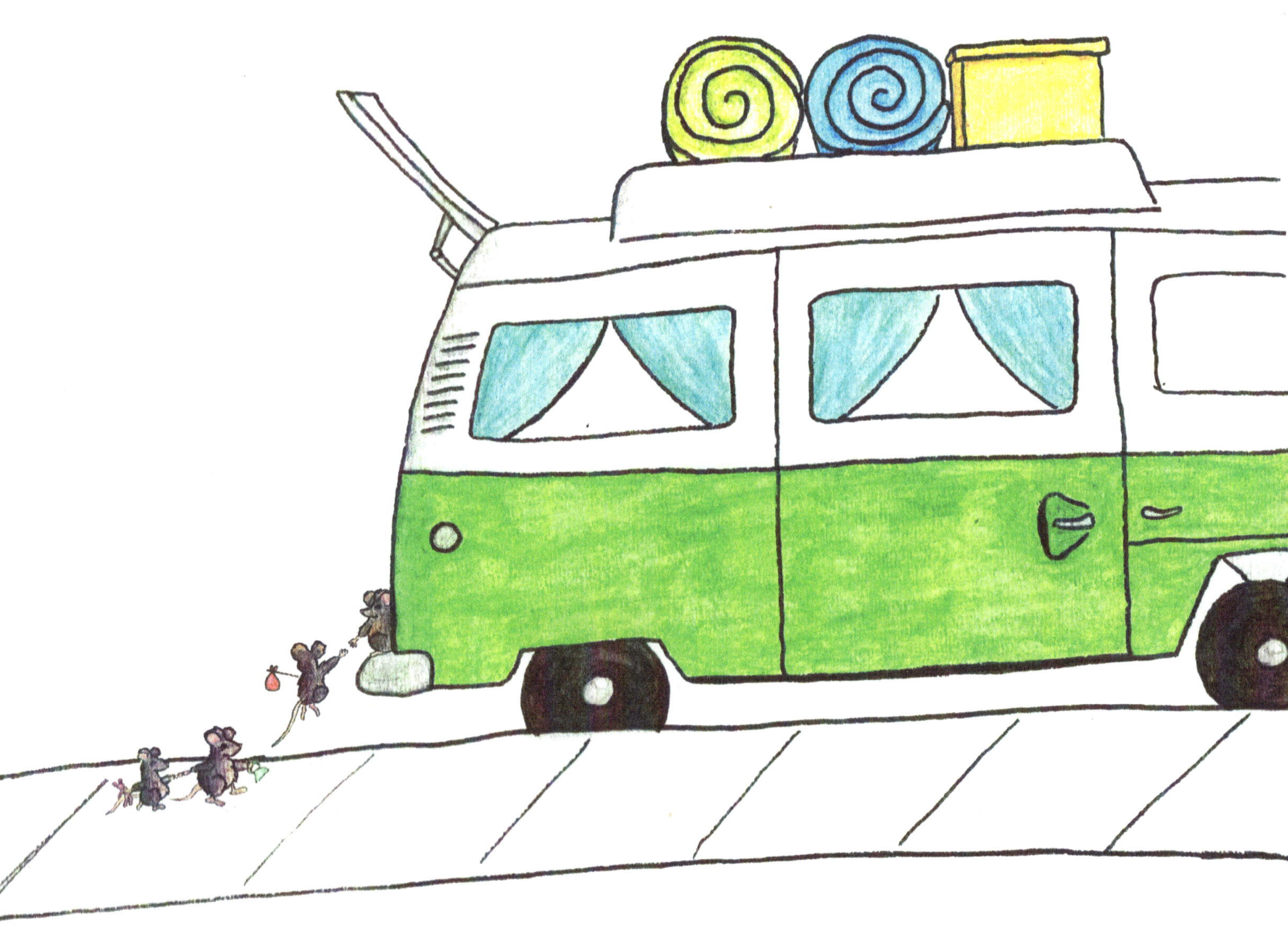

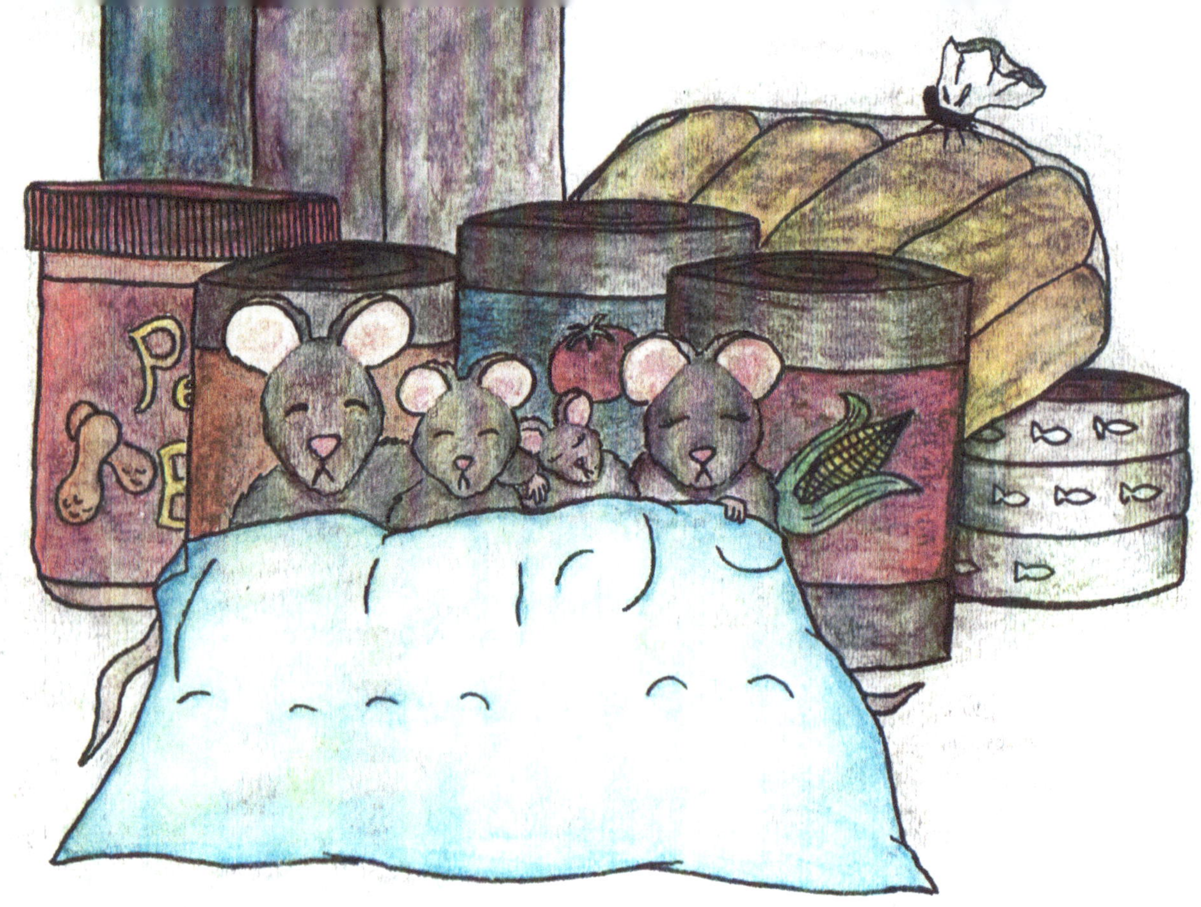

# Chapter 7

After a really long ride through the night and into the morning, the object stops moving. Snooter wakes everyone up and tells them to get ready and be quiet, as he sneaks out of the hiding place. He quickly scampers over to the hole in the door and peeks out. Wow is it bright! Squinting his eyes he jumps out. Once outside Snooter starts sniffing. Immediately he notices something quite astounding, almost too shocking for his nose! It is the air! It is so fresh and cool he feels excited and full of energy. He runs back inside to get everyone. "Come, come quick! It's amazing," says Snooter. They all come running and quickly jumped outside. Within an instant their noses are sniffing like crazy!

# Chapter 8

"Where are we?" exclaims Cattera.

"I don't know," whispers Snooter. As they walk forward the land just opens up to them and they can see waterfalls, blue lakes, and vibrant flowers. It is almost too much to take in.

Rattella looks at Cattera and starts crying, "But...sniff...sniff, where are all the other animals and where are we going to live?"

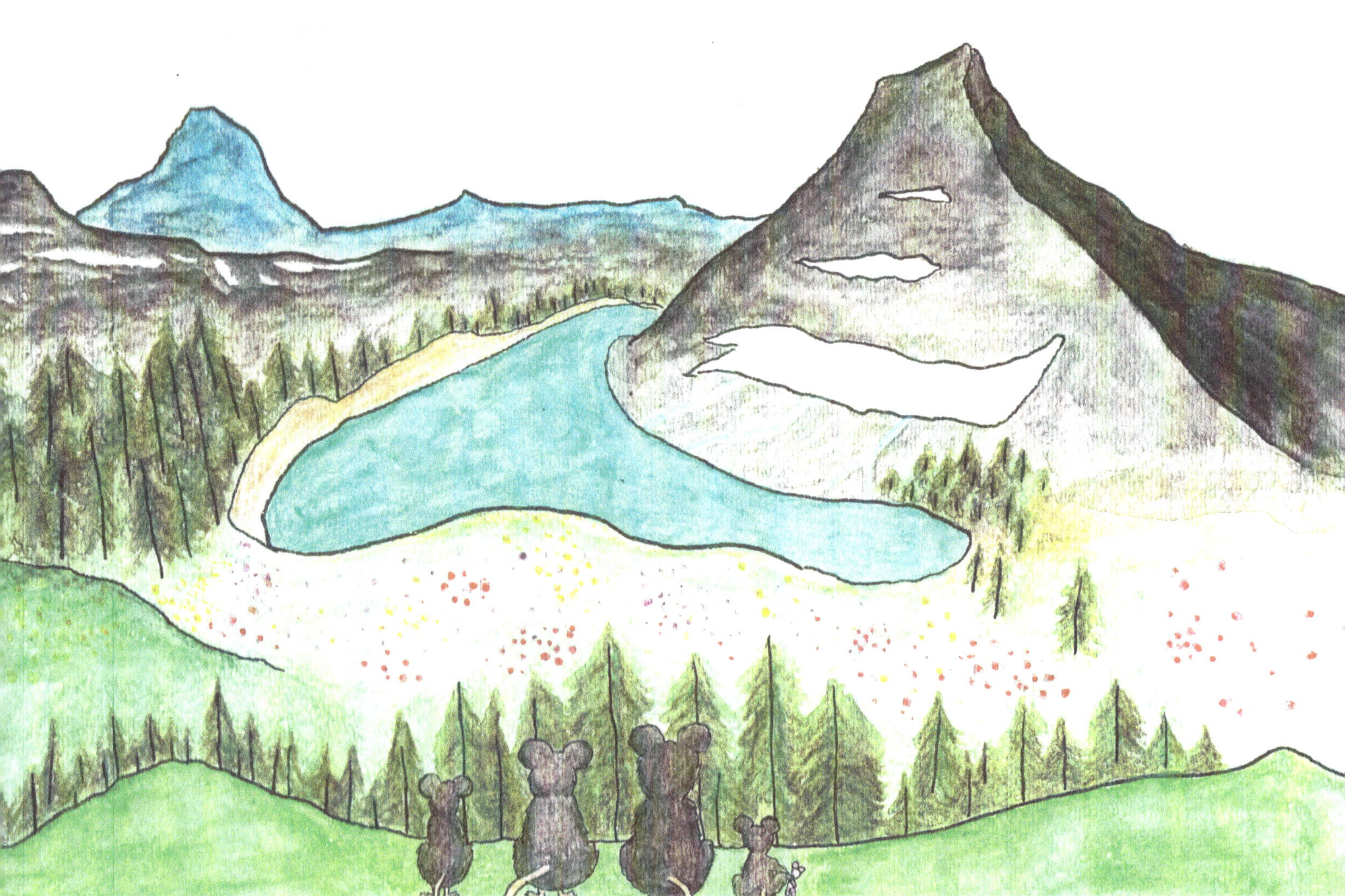

"Don't cry, honey. We just got here. We'll find a place to live today and then explore tomorrow," says Snooter with a smile and a hint of excitement.

Rooter feels so bad to see Rattella crying that he drops his head to his chest and says, "This is all my fault!" He takes off running.

"No, don't run, Rooter; you need your puffer spray!" yells Cattera. Snooter take off after him. Before you know it, Rooter starts wheezing and he can't breathe.

Snooter runs up to him and says, "Rooter, please, take a puff. This will help you breathe". Rooter grabs the puffer and takes one puff, and a second puff. Soon he starts to breathe better.

"This is not your fault, Rooter," says Cattera. "We needed to leave Smogville. We **all** were getting sick from the stinky, polluted air."

# Chapter 9

Soon enough they are all together, looking for a new rat hole. When all of a sudden Rattella yells, "Hey! I see something in the ground; come here."

"Wow," says Cattera, "look at that gigantic hole!" Sticking their noses down the hole, they can smell that no one is living there. Snooter then crawls through the hole and down the tunnel with Cattera right behind him.

"Oh my! Look at the size of this room!" Cattera says with a huge smile on her face. As they look around, they find a huge sleeping room and a massive kitchen area. They look at each other and smile.

"This will be our new home," smiles Snooter.

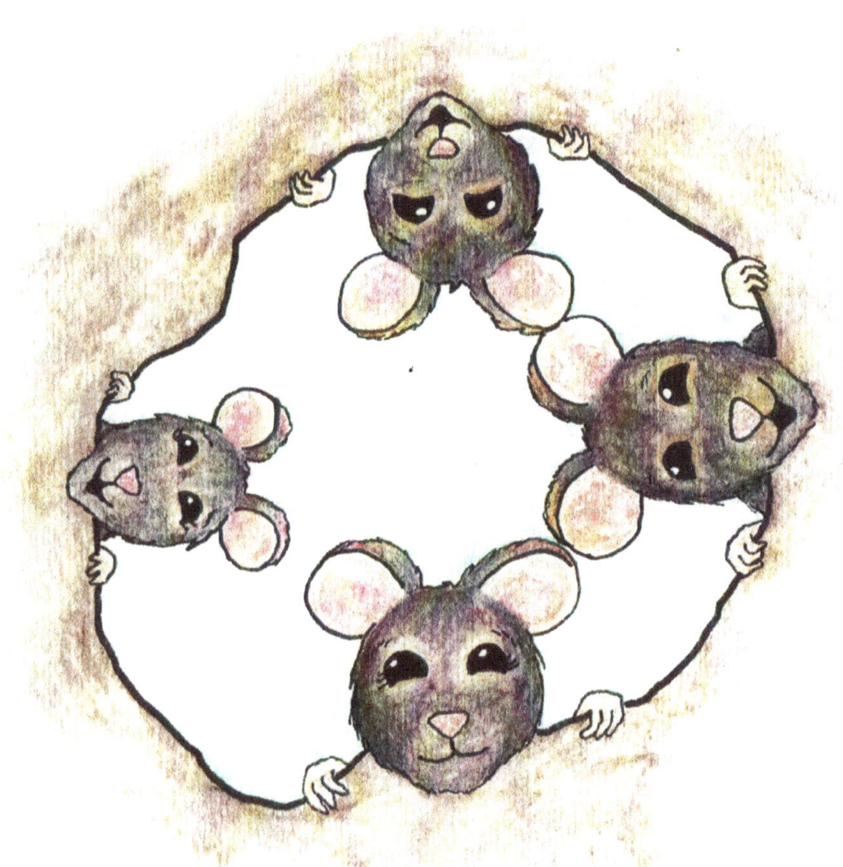

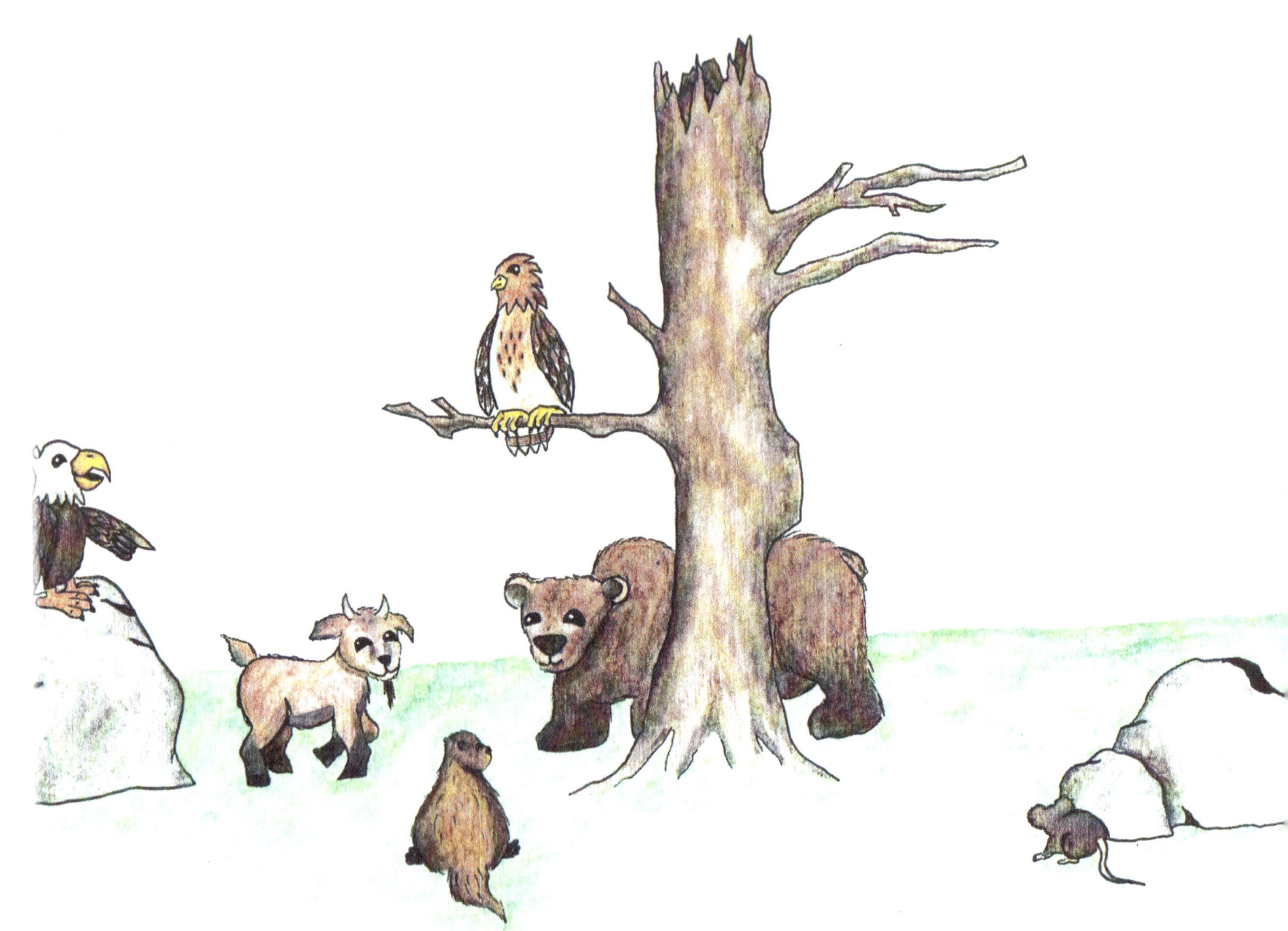

## Chapter 10

After a good night's sleep in their new home, they all got up early to go out and explore. Rooter is climbing up on a rock when he hears something. "Shhh, shhh, everyone, quiet. I hear something," Rooter says in a loud whisper. So they all drop to the ground and hide behind a rock. Snooter slowly peeks around the rock and to his amazement, he sees a bunch of animals all gathered around talking!

Then an eagle spots them and yells, "Hey what are you doing?!"

Snooter yells, "Run!!!"

Cattera hands Rooter the puffer spray, "Here take a puff; run!" They reach their new home in no time and run down the tunnel. But within minutes they hear a voice.

"Hello, is there anyone home? Please come up so I can see you," says a deep, strange voice. They all hid there with their eyes wide, looking at Snooter shaking their heads "no". He stares back and whispers, "I'm going up. You all stay here and don't make a sound!" Then he carefully climbs up through the tunnel to the opening and as he peeks out, he comes face to face with a large-looking, rat-like animal.

"Hi," the animal says. Snooter becomes so nervous that when he opens his mouth nothing comes out.

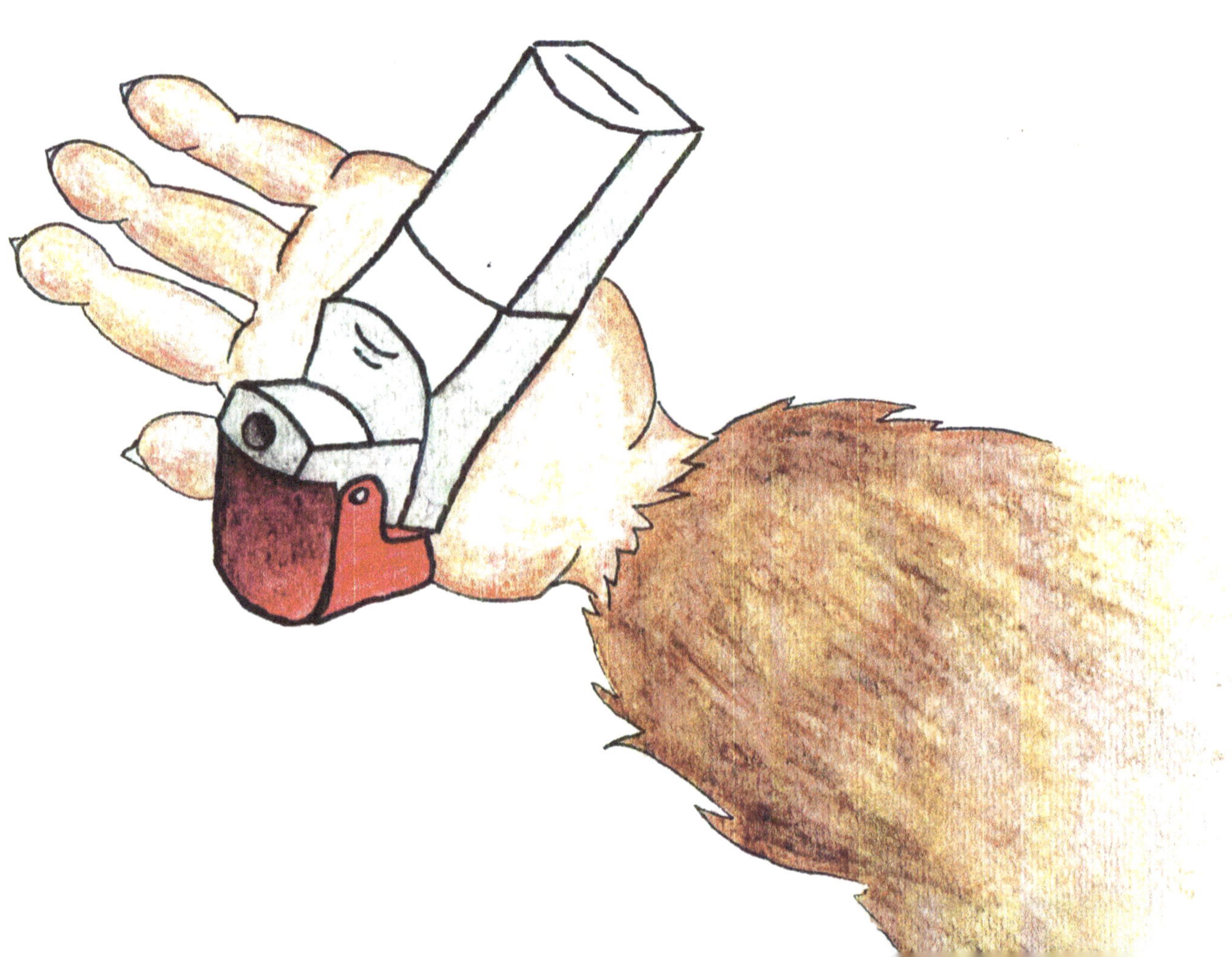

# Chapter 11

"I came to invite you to Community Night tonight, by the waterfall. Can you come?" smiles the large rat.

"Yes, umm, yes...we can, but excuse me for asking, what kind of rat are you?"

"Oh, but I'm not a rat, I'm a marmot," just then he turns and scampers away.

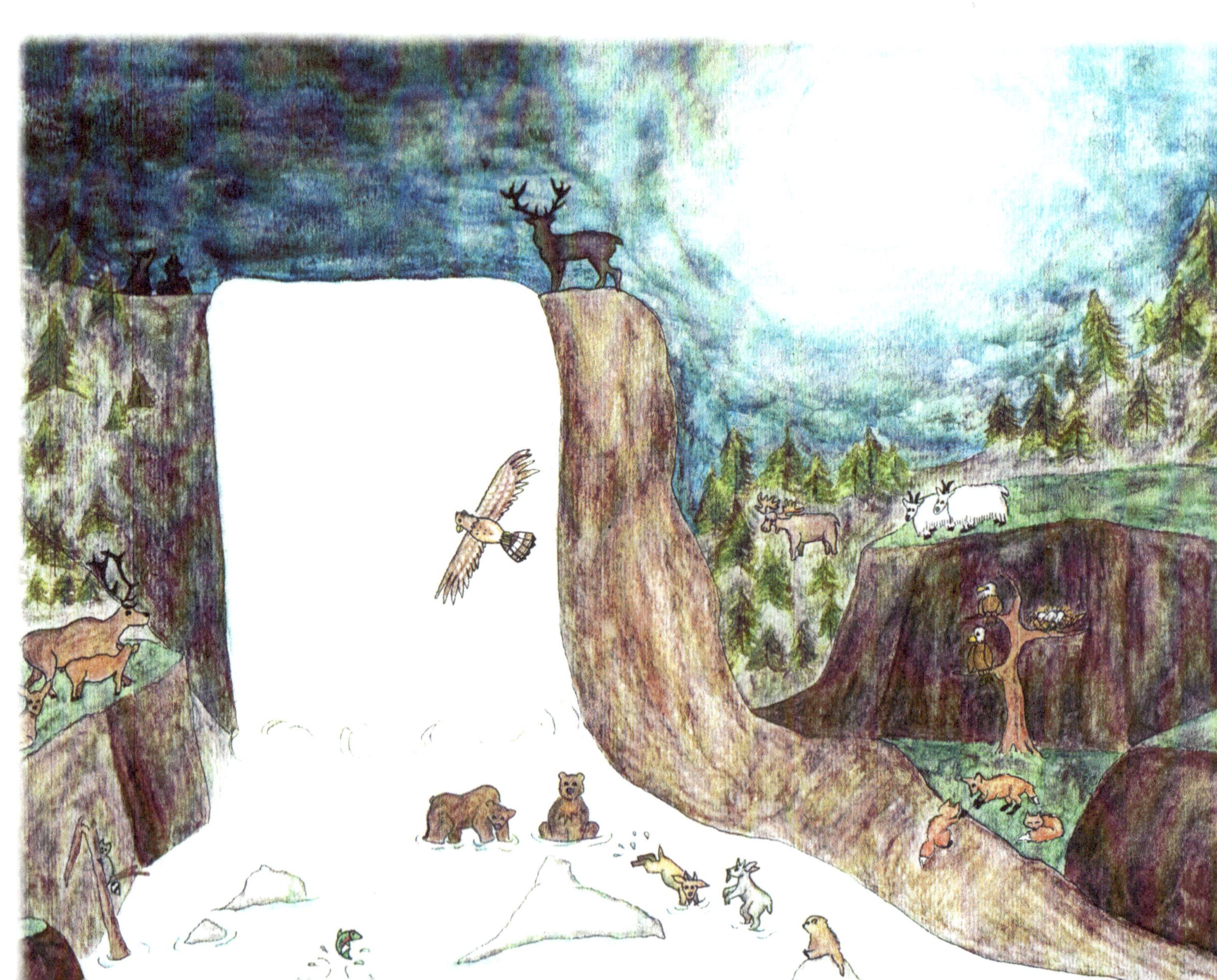

That night there is a full moon that lights up their way to the waterfall, which makes it easier to find. As they all get closer to the waterfall, they see hundreds of animals. The animals are all laughing and smiling; it is like a party! "I wonder what they are all so excited about?" says Rooter.

Just then the crowd grows silent and Marmot steps out of the crowd toward them. "Thank you for coming. We are so excited to have you join us!" He turns around and holds out his paws toward the crowd and yells, "Welcome these new friends." A huge smile pours over Cattera's face and tears well up in her eyes. The crowd cheers and the festivities begin.

# Chapter 12

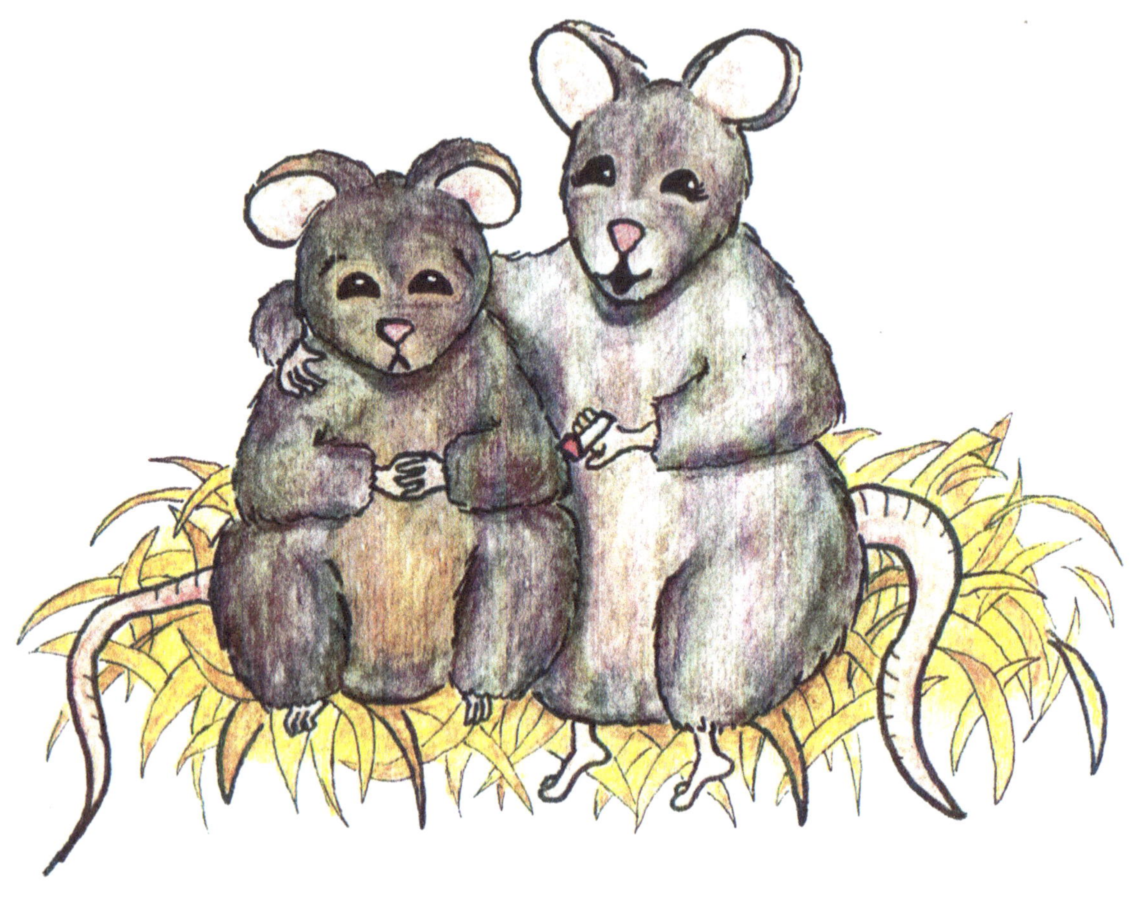

The next day Rooter goes out to play with his new friends. They are all playing a game of Hide and Seek Tag. Goatee is "It" and boy is he fast; he tagged Grizzly right away! Rooter is so excited he jumps in, running this way and that, trying not to get caught. All of a sudden he can't breathe. "Not again" thinks Rooter, not in front of my new friends! He then drops to the ground holding his chest, trying to catch his breath. Goatee runs up to Rooter to see what is happening. *"Wheeze… Please… go get my mom,"* wheezes Rooter.

Goatee looks up at the sky and yells, "Eagle, quickly fly and get Rooter's mom!"

Within minutes Cattera comes running with his puffer spray. Rooter takes a puff, and another puff. After a few minutes he feels good enough to walk. Rooter gets up feeling so embarrassed he keeps his head down so he won't have to see anyone. "Thank you," yells Cattera, "I'm taking Rooter home, and he'll be ok. Come by later if you'd like."

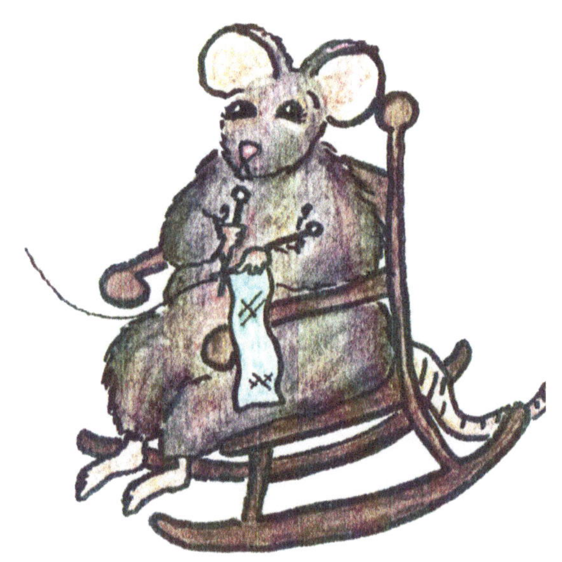

# Chapter 13

For two days Rooter just hangs around the rat hole refusing to go out and play and, most of all, see his new friends. "Rooter, this is not right. Go out and play. Just take your puffer spray with you like Dr. Puddlemug told you," Cattera says, looking at Rooter.

"I can't, everyone thinks I'm weird!" cries Rooter. Just then Rooter hears someone yelling down the hole. Rooter crawls to see Goatee standing there.

"Hi, Rooter, we came to see how you're doing," smiles Goatee. Rooter looks behind Goatee and there they are, all his friends standing there smiling at him.

"Uh...yeah...I'm doing better," Rooter says.

"Well, we all came here to tell you that there are a few of us that understand what happened to you and how you feel," Goatee says with such concern.

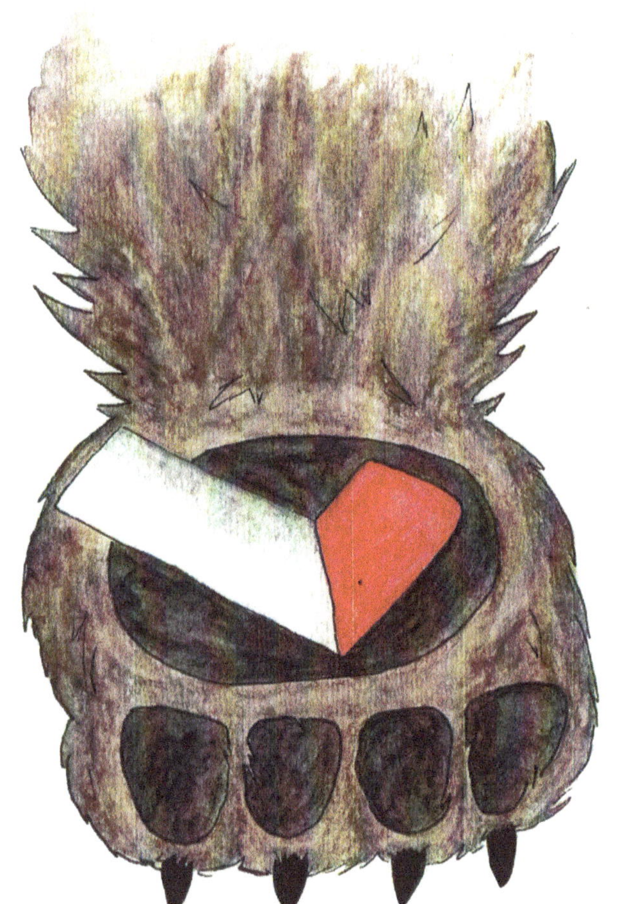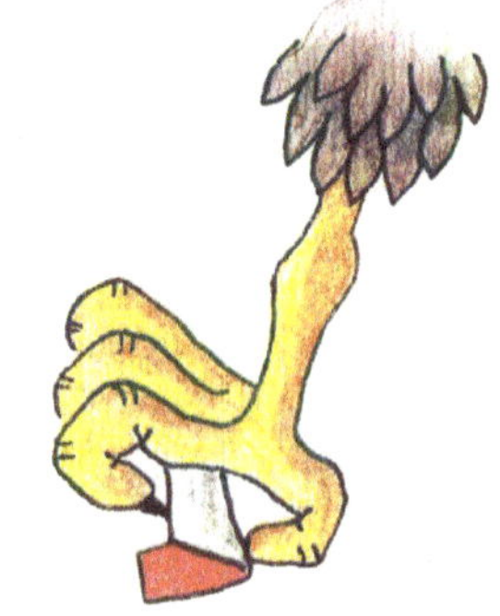

# Chapter 14

Just then Grizzly, Marmot and Eagle all step forward toward Rooter. "Rooter, we also use a puffer spray to help us breathe when we play. All three of us have asthma and we know how it feels when you can't breathe," says Grizzly.

"Uh huh, yep, sure do," they all chime in together.

"So please, Rooter, come out and play with us, but this time bring your puffer spray. We all have ours!" smiles Goatee.

Rooter has a huge smile on his face. He jumps up, grabs his puffer spray and is out the door in a flash.

Cattera watches as they head out to play. Then she yells, "Wait, Rooter, come here!"

Rooter runs back to his mom, "What, mom?"

Cattera grabs Rooter and gives him a huge hug. "Rooter, I'm so proud of you. I know you can do this, I love you!"

Rooter gives his mom a big squeeze and runs off with his friends. Life just couldn't get any better, thinks Cattera as she smiles.

The End

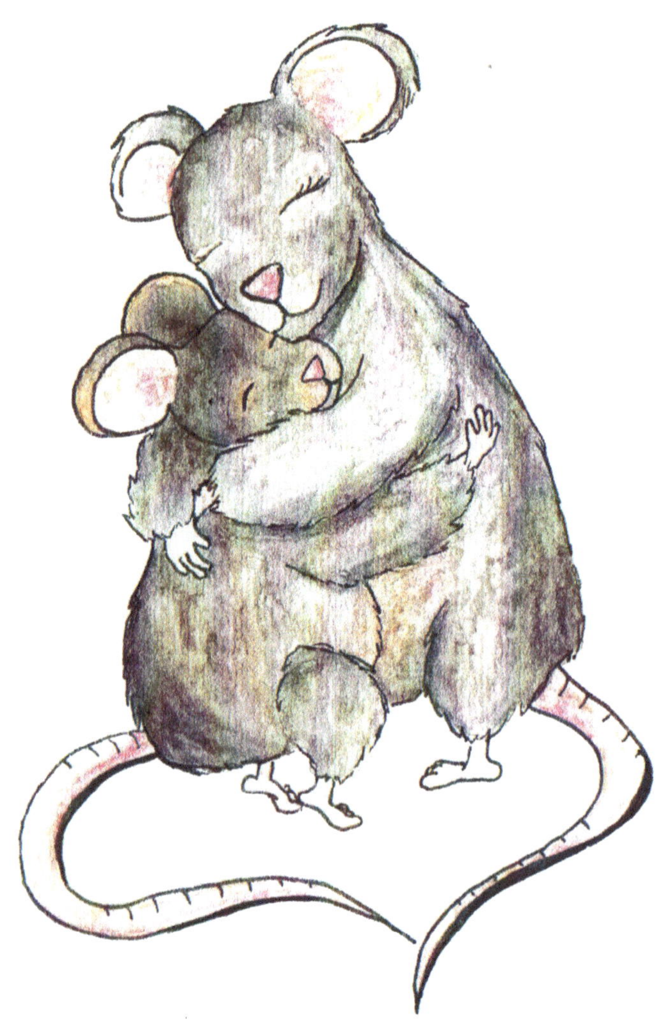

www.ingramcontent.com/pod-product-compliance
Lightning Source LLC
Chambersburg PA
CBHW040058240726
48664CB00004B/1249